The Power of Healthy Eating

"Eating Clean, Staying Lean!"

by

Teresa Giordano

www.thepoweroffitness.com

poweroffitness@comcast.net

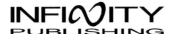
INFINITY PUBLISHING

Copyright © 2010 by Teresa Giordano

ISBN 0-7414-6202-8

Printed in the United States of America

Published August 2010

INFINITY PUBLISHING
1094 New DeHaven Street, Suite 100
West Conshohocken, PA 19428-2713
Toll-free (877) BUY BOOK
Local Phone (610) 941-9999
Fax (610) 941-9959
Info@buybooksontheweb.com
www.buybooksontheweb.com

<u>Acknowledgments</u>

I must thank quite a list of people who have made this journey for me a Success!

First, my daughter, Nikki Siske, who has helped me with the body of the book, to assure that I have the details that are necessary, and to actually get it on its way to Publishing!

My husband Richard, who has been put on the back burner for months while I worked many hours to make a dream come true.

I also want to thank my good friend Joe Cannon, who has been able to guide me to the publishing company that made my first cookbook an Actual Reality and not just a Dream.

To all of my wonderful clients who have pretty much been my "taste testers" giving me feedback and allowing me to make changes constantly to have them try again.

I also want to add that the family members who have been a part of our family gatherings for more than 24 years, who have all given me the confidence to actually write a cookbook, because they always came back for more.

I hope that you and your family enjoy as much as mine does.

About the Author

Growing up in a single parent household with a brother and a mom who worked a lot of hours so she could provide for us, it forced me into the kitchen at an early age of 10 yrs old.

I look back now and have to laugh at the many blunders that were made, and of course my brother never lets me forget one in particular. I wanted to impress my mom and I made a very big dinner of lasagna and was so proud of myself for following the directions. I went through every step thinking how it was going to be so yummy when it's done, Needless to say, it was a total disaster! I managed to mistake a block of Butter for a block of cheese. The final dish came out looking like a oil slick mess and it was not edible!

I didn't allow this disaster to keep me out of the kitchen. I have always enjoyed both cooking and cleaning. In my earlier years I managed a house cleaning business working quite long hours in order to provide for my family as well, just like my mom did.

I still found that being in the Kitchen was a comfort to me.

I began working in the Health and Fitness field when I was 29 years old, and with a constant mindset of being healthy and stronger my enthusiasm in the kitchen changed too. My Recipes began to emphasize on "healthier, cleaner eating."

Over the past 15 years I have worked with clients who are trying to make life style changes to fight health concerns such as Diabetes, high blood pressure, obesity, and heart disease. Knowing that we are what we eat, our body does respond to the good and the bad that we ingest. Working with these clients, with the passion that I have to help them be better at all that they do, I have come up with many recipes that I would like to now share.

My only hope is, if I can manage to convince you that "eating well isn't so difficult", and you can pass this message onto to your children and Grandchildren, we will soon be on the other side of this war we fight each day with our health concerns.

In Good Health, Teresa Giordano

Testimonials

For Nine years, Teresa Giordano has been guiding me with her expertise in physical fitness at her Power of Fitness studio. As a bonus I've been lucky enough to be a taste tester for many of her delicious, energy packed Recipes!

Always emphasizing on the importance of Proper nutrition in achieving a healthy lifestyle, Teresa has served up a variety of snacks and meals that have been enjoyed by myself and all of her clients. From Protein shakes, homemade bars, turkey chili, just to name a few.

As you look through these pages you will find an array of Tantalizing, healthy dishes that fit perfectly into your life changing plan towards healthy living. Bon Appétit!

Amy Kliegman

Bookstores have shelves overflowing with cookbooks ju jour.

What makes Teresa's cookbook special are these three things:

1. I am picky about flavor, texture and eye appeal and have personally sampled and endorse with both thumbs up Teresa's cooking!

2. Teresa cares about Nutrition- she is forever emailing tips, statistics and other vitals about right and wrong foods.

3. Teresa's Recipes are doable! Even people with extra crazy schedules can prepare her tested and true dishes.

Therese Long, a Fan of Teresa Giordano for over 7 years.

Speaking about her Orange Flax muffins in particular, Nutritious, delicious and filling is what makes this muffin Irresistible! It is definitely a family favorite and every time I take them to a luncheon I am asked for the recipe. Teresa's Chicken salad is awesome too!

Elaine Bassford

With Teresa's Encouragement, I have changed my eating habits. I now have a very clean diet. I have tried several of her recipes which are both satisfying and easy to prepare. Her Recipe for Braised Greens is wonderful, as is the chicken vegetable soup! I have sampled her breakfast cookies and energy pops and will certainly make those for my family in the future. I am 58 years old, and I have lost more than 20 pounds while eating healthy, delicious foods. Teresa's Recipes have taken boredom out of clean eating.

Pat- Annapolis MD.

I'm a relative newcomer to Teresa's healthy outlook on food, but in six short months she's made me a believer! Teresa's recipes are nutritious and loaded with good-for-you ingredients. If you don't know which recipe to try, start with the braised greens and sweet potatoes....easy to make and with lots of flavor. Guaranteed to warm your tummy on a cool day!

Anna

Introduction

Eating should NOT be scary

From the point of view of a personal trainer, a mom, a wife, and someone who spends each day "teaching" clients how to eat as well as the benefits of "movement every single day".

When it comes to weight loss so often I encounter the client who pretty much has a very complicated and confusing relationship with food.

I begin our session with the request of a 3 day journal of everything they eat as well as activity which allows me to guide them into a healthier daily routine.

Sometimes it requires what I call a "cleansing eating plan" that typically will be a week long. This encourages the toxic build up that is what is causing them to feel so sluggish and not burn calories in a more efficient manner.

It doesn't mean they are on a "liquid diet" it simply focuses on "clean eating", high water content foods, no sugar, no caffeine, no salt.

They are astonished after a week that they are not only thinking clearer, sleeping better, have more energy, and they've lost a few lbs. of bloat! Yes it's typically water weight at first but you shouldn't be discouraged by this.

The weight on the scale should be the weight of your muscle, tissue and water and fat. The number on the scale is NOT what you judge your fitness level by. You eliminate toxins, water retention, allowing you to workout harder and longer and feed your muscle good quality protein, fueling your body with high fiber carbohydrates that will allow you to continue to be on your journey to a healthier "YOU"!

This book was not meant to be a "diet". I prefer to refer to it as a teaching guide to help you along the way in your Journey.

My goal is to help you understand that living a healthy lifestyle is not as complicated as many believe and eating healthy is NOT as difficult as one may think.

I talk to my clients daily about making "simple quick" meals that taste good and allow you more time to be with family and friends and you will continue to feel your BEST.

Contents

Pump Up with Beverly

Quick Fixins

Tips from the Author

QUICK BREAKFAST WITH BALANCED NUTRIENTS

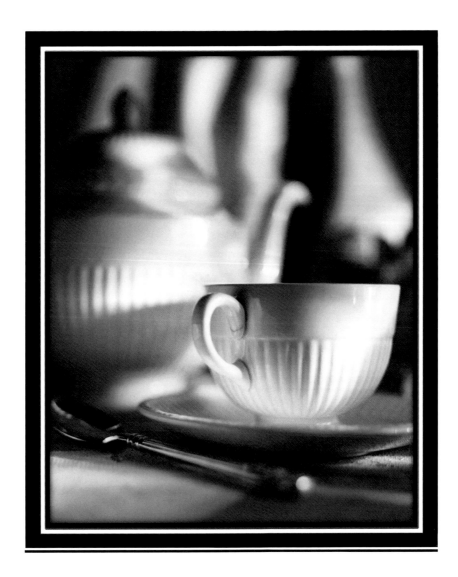

Coconut oil and coconut milk have received a bad reputation over the years. Coconut oil in moderation can help you shed belly fat. It's great for high heat cooking in a sauté pan and low fat coconut milk can make a great substitute for lactose intolerance.

In addition **Greek Yogurt Plain** is an important part of your diet because it packs a punch with CLA (conjugated linoleic acid) which helps fight fat. It has the highest amount of protein and lowest amount of sugar when it comes to yogurt.

OAT TORTILLA FOR THE TRUE CLEAN EATER

(of course great for everyone)

1/2 cup oat flour
1/2 cup raw oat bran
1 cup just egg whites
1/3 c water
2 Tbsp. grape seed or coconut oil

Mix all ingredients in blender. Batter will be thin. Heat a non stick skillet and pour about 1/4 c into hot skillet. As soon as tiny bubbles appear, flip. It should be very light brown toasted on the side cooking cook about 1.5-2 minute per side

Note: this is a very clean eating tortilla. You can make wraps, top it with nut butter and eat as is. Or use it as your toast for eggs! They can be cooled and wrapped individually to freeze, or plate them in the refrigerator to eat within 3 days. (I would recommend toasting them lightly the next day before eating)

GREEK YOGURT PARFAIT

6 oz of Greek 2% fat plain yogurt

1 Tablespoon raw or roasted unsalted pumpkin seeds or walnuts

1 T chai seed (antioxidant rich omega 3)

1/4 c. Fresh berries

Starting with the yogurt, layer your parfait and enjoy. Make ahead for the busy morning rush!

Calories: 190 Fat: healthy fats 3.5 grams protein: 16 grams carbs 9 grams (from fruits and high fiber chia)

Note: make this even more filling and fiber rich by adding 1/3 c Fiber one cereal on top! I prefer to use 2% fat yogurt and add healthier fats to this Parfait ** this is also a great choice after a workout to replenish your body. Chia seed is rich in antioxidants, fiber and a must to incorporate each day.

SIMPLE OVER EASY EGGS ATOP BRAN MUFFIN

(balance of fiber protein and healthy fat)

1 VitaTop multiBran muffin toasted (100 calories for the top only)
1 whole egg + 2 egg whites
1 spray of canola spectrum for pan
1 Tbsp. natural nut butter of your choice

While the muffin top is toasting, cook 1 whole egg and 2 egg whites in a hot skillet. Once the whites are cooked flip it and take it off heat. Spread 1 Tablespoon Natural nut butter on top and top it with your eggs.

Serves 1. calories 280 Protein: 18 grams carbs: 25 high fiber energy Fiber:8 grams

Note: This quick breakfast is a staple for me on early mornings when I know I need quality fiber and protein to get me through the morning. I often will make the exact Recipe but use Eziekel English muffin only 1/2 toasted.

FRESH ORANGE CHIA SEED BRAN MUFFIN

1 C raw oat bran

1 C king Arthur whole wheat flour

1/2 C chia goodness (www.ruthshempfoods.com)

1 C raw natural wheat bran

1 T baking powder

1 tsp. baking soda

1/2 c organic brown sugar

1 C low fat buttermilk

1/2 c Safflower oil (high antioxidants) or canola oil

2 whole organic large eggs

1 large fresh orange washed and chopped in food processor

5 pitted chopped prunes

In large bowl combine oat bran, flour ,chia goodness, wheat bran, baking powder and baking soda. mix well. In Food Processor Bowl combine the chopped orange with rind & prunes, brown sugar, buttermilk, oil, and eggs. puree leaving orange chunks. Pour wet ingredients into dry and mix well. Use a 1/4 cup measuring out into muffin pan. Bake 375' 15-18 minutes.

Makes 15 Muffins. Calories: 240 protein: 7 grams fiber: 6.5 grams carbs: 26 grams

Note: I like to use rubber bake wear for easy release. Remember your breakfast should be at least 300 calories and this muffin is packed with fiber! I have been known as the muffin lady for years. This one makes you feel like you are cheating because they are so yummy! Great for breakfast on the run!

EASY BRAN MUFFIN WITH A LITTLE HELP

(Tweaking a boxed muffin mix no one will ever know)

1 box Hodgson mill Bran muffin mix 7 oz
1 T canola oil
1/2 c plain rice dream (dairy substitute)
1 small Zucchini grated
1/4 c all whites egg whites
1/3 c mini organic dark chocolate chips

Preheat oven 400. I like to use rubber muffin pans non stick, however use spectrum organic non toxic spray if using metal. Mix all of the ingredients in a large bowl. Let sit for about 5 min. begin to scoop about 1/4 c mixture into each muffin cup bake 10-12 minutes

Note: everyone knows I am the muffin lady :) and make tons of them, but when unexpected company comes these are easy to have ready with a cup of coffee or tea and they're healthy! You can adjust the recipe with shredded carrots, raisins nuts etc.

HIGH FIBER MOIST BRAN MUFFIN

(make ahead and freeze)

1 C raw organic sugar
1/2 c canola oil
1/2 c Greek 0% fat plain yogurt
1 whole egg + 4 egg whites
1 T. baking soda
1 T fresh ground cinnamon
1 tsp sea salt
1 10 oz can fruit cocktail undrained but Low in sugar
3.5 c whole wheat flour
1/2 C almond meal ground
1 quart low fat buttermilk
1 15 oz box Kelloggs complete oat bran cereal flakes
1/2 c golden raisins
1/2 c finely chopped walnuts

Combine all ingredients in a very large bowl. I use a wooden spoon to mix cereal in last with the raisins and nuts. Beat the rest together to combine. Spoon into muffin tins (I like using rubber cups to prevent sticking and toxins in my food) * if not using rubber, make sure you spray spectrum canola w/ flour into each tin. Fill about 2/3 full and bake at 400 for 15 min. ovens are different so watch them and make sure they are baked through but not dry.

Note: These are wonderful when having a brunch. You can keep a bowl in refrigerator up to 3 days and bake as you want them or Freeze.
Makes approx. 48 muffins depending on size of cup.

PEACH MANGO SHAKE

(Shake for anytime, but perfect for a hot summer day!)

2/3 c frozen or Fresh in season peaches
2/3 c frozen mango
1 T honey or Agave

6 oz of plain greek yogurt *use either 2% fat or 0%*
1 Tablespoon Flax oil or Udo oil
Optional 1 scoop Beverly vanilla UMP protein powder

Calories without Protein: 184 protein 4 grams fiber 2.4 grams carbs 44 grams Calories with Protein added: 294 (this is a meal) Protein with added: 24 grams fiber 2.4 grams carbs:45g.

Note: This section of shakes you can make it a meal by adding your Beverly protein powder, or you can keep it light as a refreshing snack. I always keep frozen fruit to make it easy but there is nothing better than a fresh peach when they're in season!

CARROT CAKE PANCAKES

(Best to make on the weekend, not as quick preparing)

1 C oat flour + 1/4 c almond meal
1/4 c slightly toasted walnuts chopped fine
2 Teasp. baking powder
1 T cinnamon
1/2 tsp fresh ground nutmeg
dash cloves
dash ginger
1/3 c organic brown sugar
3/4 c low fat buttermilk (or use light coconut milk if you are dairy free)
1 T canola oil
1 1/2 tsp high quality vanilla
2 egg whites + 1 whole egg
2 large carrots peeled washed and finely grated

Mix flours and next 7 ingredients thru ginger. In separate bowl, combine brown sugar, and next 4 ingredients fold in carrots and combine the two bowls to make a batter. Spray skillet with spectrum non chemical spray and use 1/4 cup batter per pancake. On medium heat cook about 1 min each side. It's ok if they are damp on top as you will toast the leftover for another day. *treat drizzle 1/4 T. only organic honey or 1/4 tsp. natural nut butter.

Serving 2 mini pancakes: 63 calories 5 g. fiber

Note: I made this treat during a very long winter stuck in the house but wanting to still eat healthy. You can individually wrap them once they've cooled, place in freezer bag and take out as you want. Toast them on medium or microwave in paper towel for 30 seconds, than drizzle with honey. Yes this is a higher carb treat but all very natural good carbs.

BLACKBERRY BANANA SMOOTHIE

(Helps melt belly fat)

2 C fresh or frozen blueberries
1 small banana
1/2 C light coconut milk
1/2 c plain low fat greek yogurt (if off dairy add 1 T flax or udo oil)
1 T fresh lemon juice + 1 t Zest of lemon
1 T organic honey or agave
3 ice cubes

Place all in blender puree. Serves 2. If you are alone cut all ingredients in half.

Per serving 250 calories 5 grams healthy fats 6 grams protein with yogurt 9 g. fiber

Note: Adding healthy fats into your day in moderation help flush fat. Coconut milk and coconut oil have received a bad reputation over the years. It's great for high heat cooking and low fat coconut milk makes a great substitute for lactose intolerance!

Appetizers

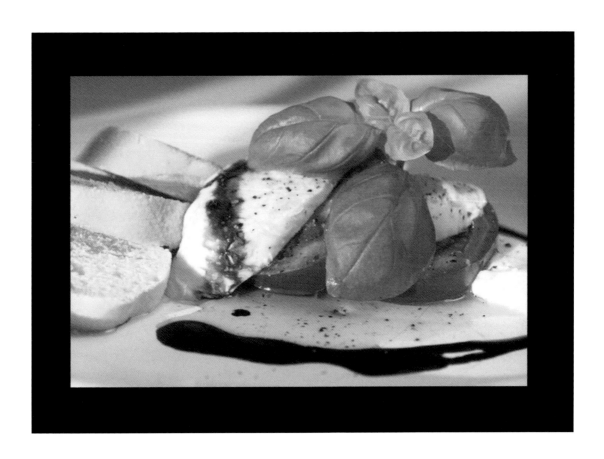

BAKED KALE CHIPS

Large bag of triple washed cut up Kale
spritz of olive oil
Sea salt 1 tsp.

Simply lay out kale on a large baking tray. Spritz it with olive oil and sea salt bake at 375 approx 10 minutes to crisp crunch you may want to shake the dish half way or use tongs to move the kale around to assure equal crispness.

Note: This is one of the easiest healthy ways to get your friends and family to skip the high fat chips. Kale is nutrient rich and good for you. YOU will be amazed at how much you will enjoy this one! *you can add hot pepper flakes or NO sodium seasoning to adjust to your taste. *allow to sit and air dry to keep crisp don't cover right away.

FRITTATA

(your choice what meal?)

1/2 c chopped sweet peppers (jar roasted peppers drained are even faster)
3 T finely chopped sweet onion
4- roma tomatoes chopped in 1/2 or diced
1 whole egg + 6 egg whites (1 cup)
black Pepper
fresh oregano
parmesan cheese, feta cheese or goat cheese 1 Tablespoon

Preheat oven 375 In med. skillet that is oven proof spritz with spectrum organic spray add peppers and onion sauté for 5 minutes. Add 4 roma tomatoes chopped or diced. Spread mixture evenly on bottom of pan use fork to mix whole egg and egg whites. Pour over the top of mixture in pan that is still on heat, sprinkle with pepper oregano and your choice of cheese. Place in the oven for 10 minutes until top is done.

Add in's: *you can use roasted peppers instead of tomato zucchini or spinach as your green vegetable making sure the zucchini is cooked with the onion and peppers.

140 calories per serving 115 Protein: 9 grams fat: 6 grams 3 grams fiber with green vegetable added in

Note: It's NOT necessary to add salt when you are adding cheese. If eating at dinner serve with a nice green salad.

DEVILED EGGS WITH A OMEGA PUNCH

12 hard boiled eggs cooled
2 avocado inside scooped out
1 tbsp. extra virgin olive oil
1 tsp paprika
1 Tbsp. finely chopped Red onion
1 drop Tabasco *optional*
1 dash sea salt and black pepper

Remove yolk from eggs (use for another time) smash avocado gently adding the rest of ingredients scooping or using a pastry bag fill each hardboiled egg white with the mixture. This makes a great appetizer and is filled with clean protein and healthy omega fats.

CHICKEN SALAD STUFFED TOMATO

4 plum or small roma tomatoes cut top off and de-seed
1/2 c of my recipe chicken salad
2 T fresh cut chives
1 T paprika

After washing and cleaning out inside of tomato, stand them up on a serving platter, scoop a heaping tablespoon of chicken salad into each sprinkle with chives and paprika ** for Vegetarians use a combination of 1% fat whipped cottage cheese mixed with golden Raisins instead*

Calories 51 per stuffed tomato bite 4 g carbs 2 gram fat

Note: I have made a large platter with both displayed to please the crowd and it's nice to pick up and eat without worrying about having utensils.

ROASTED EDAMAME

Preheat oven 400.

Toss 1 lb frozen edamame that has been thawed with 1/2 tsp. sea salt. *it's important to stay strict on the amount of salt we use*

1 tablespoon olive oil

You want to roast for at least 30 min. if you have a convection oven. Stir half way thru roasting process.

1/4 cup serving = 130 cal. and 2 g fiber

STUFFED SWEET PEPPER OR STUFFED ITALIAN TOMATO

Prepare stuffing:
In bowl combine
1 T Crème Frese
1/3 c 1% fat whipped cream cheese
1 medium size sweet cucumber finely chopped and peeled.

Cut the tops off of the small tomato clean out the center well wash and dry
Use 1 T of filling in each one.

Using sweet long red chili pepper cut down the center, and clean out inside
Using 1 T filling to stuff

*These make great snacks during parties or entertaining without the guilt.

GARLIC SHRIMP APPETIZER:

1 lb peeled and deveined shrimp, toss in large bowl with 1/3 c olive oil
1 whole lemon squeezed and 3 T fresh zest
1/4 tsp sea salt 1/4 c fresh parsley

Mix it all up and set aside covered for about 30 min. or in Refrigerator for a few hours

On either an indoor grill or outdoor hot grill, place the shrimp on grill tray so it doesn't fall through, and cook about 30-45 seconds if grill is very hot. Turn and repeat. Place the shrimp in a serving platter.

Meanwhile place a good quality French bread slice that was drizzled with a touch of olive oil on the hot grill. Just for 10 seconds to toast. On top of each slice of bread, place 1/2 T soft goat cheese and then place 2 shrimp on top of that.

Delicious and everyone wants more!

ITALIAN APPETIZER PIZZA BITES

Being married to an Italian and following the normal entertaining protocol, When your company arrives they should have plenty of bite size appetizers to graze on until dinner is ready. This one was a favorite of my step sons in the past, as well as my dear late Father n law, who could make a meal out of this and a big glass of red wine. :)

Middle Eastern Flat bread
*depending on how many you want to serve, separate and place on a cookie sheet, spray a touch of olive oil on them and toast in an oven for 5 minutes

Meanwhile get your toppings ready so you can get it right back into the oven.

Toppings:
1 pint grape tomatoes
1 can drained artichoke hearts
*both of these are tossed with a touch of olive oil and than also put into the oven to wilt about 5 minutes.
1T finely grated Fresh parmesan cheese
2 C spinach or arugula
1/2 c left over boiled chicken breast (I like using organic free range)
1 whole shredded green zucchini
1 T olive oil
black pepper (optional red pepper flakes)
fresh basil and oregano
3 T total of soft goat cheese or use tiny balls of mozzarella cheese

Once the flat bread is out of oven, top each one with a small amount of tomatoes, artichoke hearts that have been roasting, zucchini, goat cheese, basil, spinach or arugula, oregano, pepper and pulling the chicken breast apart making shreds, lay on top. Drizzle with olive oil and a sprinkle of fresh parmesan cheese and place back into the oven for only about 5 min. or so to allow everything to melt together.

Use a sharp long knife or pizza cutter and cut these into two or even four. Place them on a serving platter and they will disappear!

The calories of course depend on how much of everything you add but approximately for 1/2 of each flat bread: calories 160   fiber 5 grams

SOUP AND SALAD

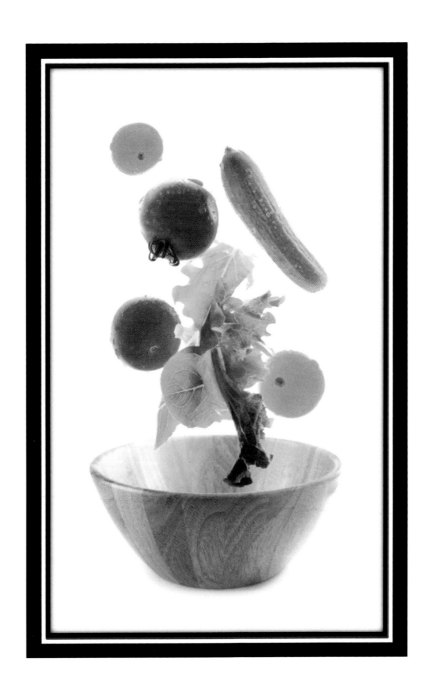

BETTER SIDE OF CABBAGE SLAW

(cookouts or anytime)

1 cup finely shredded carrots
2 C purple and green combined cabbage chopped into small pieces washed
1/3 c plain 0% fat Greek yogurt
1/3 c. light mayo
1T celery seed
1 T white champagne vinegar
1 teaspoon organic raw sugar
1 T black pepper and 1/2 tsp sea salt
1/4 c organic dried cranberries
1/4 c slivered raw almonds

Combine the yogurt and all ingredients the down to (and including) almonds in large bowl. Mix well and add cabbage and carrots. Stir and cover refrigerate until ready to serve.

<u>Note:</u> Do to mixing 0% fat yogurt with the light mayo it eliminates some of the fat, but also adds in calcium and extra shot of protein. This is a very light side dish that will compliment cookouts or anytime you are in a rush for dinner.

SPLIT PEA SOUP

Mix of yellow and green split peas about 35 grams total dry

3 slices cooked turkey bacon drained
1 large carrot chopped
2 garlic cloves chopped even better roasted
2 32 oz size low sodium chicken broth (you can use vegetable broth)
1 3/4 cup split peas rinsed well and drained
2 sticks of fresh rosemary
1/4 tsp sea salt and 1 T pepper
1 small sweet onion finely chopped

Sauté the bacon until crisp in a large soup pot. Remove and dry. In same pan add onion, carrot garlic and sauté for about 5 minutes. Add broth and peas and the rosemary. Bring to boil reduce heat and simmer for 2 hours. In the last 20 min. of cooking add the chopped bacon into pot, salt pepper and use a masher to mash gently some of the beans makes 4 meal size portions or 6 appetizer size

Meal size calories 150 protein 10 grams carbs: 20 grams (high fiber carbs) Fiber 10 grams

Note: I put this one under appetizer because I often serve it with our turkey burger and it's our high fiber vegetable with the meal, however you can have it as your meal and keep it lighter. For vegetarians substitute a soy based meat for flavoring.

ITALIAN WEDDING SOUP

(Not your traditional high sodium)

1 lb ground chicken breast very lean
1 egg
2 T chopped fresh parsley
1 T finely chopped sweet onion
1 garlic clove chopped
2 T high quality fresh parmesan cheese
1/4 teaspoon sea salt and 1 t black pepper
2 stalks celery chopped
1 more clove garlic chopped
1 Tbsp. good olive oil
6 cups of low sodium chicken stock
1 head Escarole chopped and washed
1/4 c grated fresh parmesan cheese

Mix together ground chicken breast, egg, parsley, sweet onion, garlic, parmesan cheese salt and pepper. Make tiny little meatballs. sauté them in a medium size skillet on med/low. (They will cook fast so only for about 3 min.) Meanwhile in a large stock pot with olive oil, sauté celery, garlic and escarole for about 2 min. adding stock pepper salt and add the meatballs into soup. Simmer about 10-15 min. as you serve sprinkle with 1 T each serving parmesan cheese.

Note: Being married to an Italian with an amazing mother n law who seriously would be offended if you didn't eat her food, I took her recipe and cut the carbs, the fat, and made this Italian favorite a bit healthier. I have in the winter, added a small amount of Barilla plus high fiber macaroni noodles to this but, with each person adding only 1/3 cup per bowl.

ASPARAGUS SOUP

14 oz low sodium chicken or vegetable broth
4 Cups water
1 yukon gold potato peeled and washed
1 shallot thinly sliced
1 clove garlic
1/2 tsp. Marjoram spice
Pinch sea salt
12 asparagus spheres washed trimmed and slices into 1" pieces
1 Tbsp. coconut milk light or evaporated skim milk

Optional- leave out 1 oz chopped Prosciutto for vegetarian version.

Place all ingredients into a large stock pot simmer for 10 minutes. Take off heat and let cool for about 10 min. Place into a blender and Puree. Place back into the stove and add the Prosciutto (if using).

Serves 4 adult size servings as an appetizer or side with Salad Calories: 174 Fat: 3 grams Carbs: 25 grams fiber 3 grams

Note: I have used turkey bacon in place of prosciutto and it's just as good with less sodium, I also have added 1 tbsp. Greek yogurt to the top when serving. My husband likes adding Tabasco sauce.

COLORFUL SALAD WITH A TWIST

(Family Favorite)

One 3.8 oz can sliced black olives drained
One 14 oz can artichoke hearts in water drained
3 large Heirloom colorful tomatoes (cut into chunks)
1/4 lb Fresh packed firm mozzarella cheese cut into bite size
1/4 c Dried Cranberries
1/4 c shelled Pistachios
2 T dried oregano
handful of Fresh basil
3 T champagne Vinaigrette
1 tsp sea salt and black pepper
3 T extra virgin olive oil

In a low rimmed, large serving bowl, Mix all of the ingredients together, stir gently allowing all of the nutritious ingredients and colors to show. This dish is not only very pretty & presents itself well, you can simply eat as is or place on top of a bed of baby spinach leaves.

Serves 4 calories 225 fat 5 grams healthy fats carbs 10 grams fiber 3 grams protein 4 grams

Note: I use this always in the spring summer for entertaining

GREEN SOUP WITH SWEET POTATO

2 T olive oil
2 small sweet onion
A dash of sea salt
1 very large organic sweet potato/yam peeled and chopped
3.5 c water
2 T fresh chopped Sage or dash of ground sage
1 large bunch kale washed and chopped
1 large bunch chard washed and chopped
5 cloves garlic peeled
3 c organic vegetable broth
Black pepper to taste and fresh squeeze of lemon

Heat in small pot- olive oil, onion, and pinch of salt, turn down heat and let sweat and sweeten 10-15 min. Meanwhile In large stock pot add sweet potato, 3.5 c water, a dash of salt, and sage- bring to boil. Lower heat and simmer 15 min. add kale and chard that have been washed and trimmed, also add garlic and vegetable broth. Simmer for 20 minutes. Add the onion to this soup mix, stir well, remove from heat to cool slightly and then Puree in blender in batches. Be careful not to fill the blender to the top. When serving you can squeeze lemon juice on top.

Note: Perfect winter soup full of B & C vitamins and minerals. Boots your immune system because it protects your Thymus (the major gland of our Immune System)

FULL OF NUTRITION CREAMY VEGETABLE SOUP

In a large stock pot
Add 1 T extra virgin olive oil
2 cloves garlic
1 cleaned and chopped leak
2 cleaned and chopped Parsnips
4 yukon gold potatoes skin on but clean and cut into large chunks
2 cleaned and chopped Carrots
1 Can drained and rinsed white Beans such as Cannellini

Add 1 large container of low sodium organic vegetable broth
2 Cups water
Simmer for about 30 minutes.

Take off heat and let cool a little so that you can place in batches into a blender and blend to a smooth texture pouring back into the pot.

Turn heat back on to low, add 1/2 cup organic coconut milk, A pinch of sea salt, 1 tsp fresh nutmeg, and dash of pepper.

Serve with a salad if you are eating vegetarian, have alone as a meal, or have as a appetizer alongside a turkey burger from my recipes!

add on's following your dietary needs you can add 1 tsp crème fresh or 1 T. Greek yogurt on top.

WHITE BEAN AND KALE SOUP

I love eating with the season, knowing that each ingredient is fresh and at its highest nutritional value.

In a large stock pot, use your spray bottle of olive oil to spray the pan, add 1 small chopped up sweet onion, and cook about 8 minutes. then add:

3 C fresh chopped Kale
1 Large washed, peeled and chopped into small pieces, Yam
1T red wine vinegar
1 bay leaf
1 T paprika
2 (15 oz cans) organic Great Northern beans rinsed (keep 1/2 cup out)
2 containers (4 cups) organic low sodium Vegetable broth

Once your soup has blended well and simmered about 15 minutes, Place the 1/2 cup beans that were kept out into a food processor or blender, add 1/4 c water and puree, pouring that mixture into your soup pot and stir.

At the end, I like to add 2 slices of already cooked chopped turkey bacon to enhance to flavor

Keeping the bacon out allows this to be vegetarian. Serves 6
Per serving 170 calories, 9 grams protein, 34 g carbs , 10 grams fiber

TEA TIME FOR ME

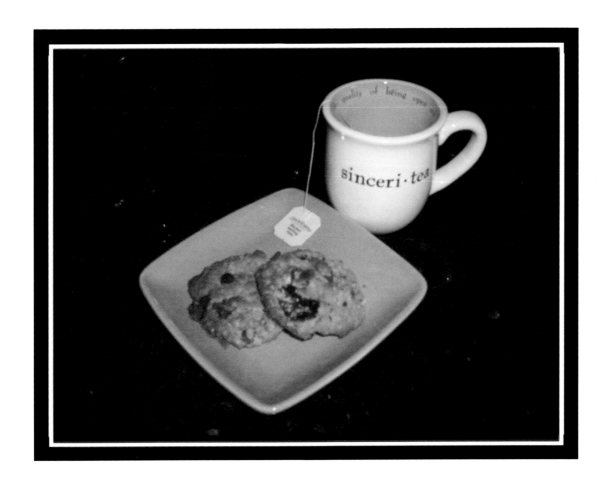

NO GUILT COOKIES

(a family favorite)

1 C organic raisins
1 stick unsalted butter
1/2 c brown sugar
3 egg whites
1/2 cup rice milk original unsweetened
2 C whole wheat flour
1 T baking powder
1 C McCains Irish oats
1 C raw oat bran
1/3 c Anutra better than flax meal (whole foods or Vitamin Shoppe)
1 T cinnamon
1/3 c raw pumpkin seeds

In large bowl combine butter, brown sugar, cream in the egg whites, and rice milk. In separate bowl combine all dry ingredients than pour into the wet Ingredient bowl. Mix on low, stir in the pumpkin seeds and Raisins Bake 375 degrees 9 min. using small cookie scoop making 30-35 cookies packed with 4 grams of fiber per cookie!

Note: my high fiber cookies can be eaten at breakfast with yogurt or even eggs as they typically are not meant to be sweet. The goal is to get your fiber in. All of them go great with tea or coffee and to encourage kids to try them you can always add chocolate chips

DATE NUT BARS

(Healthy quick make ahead snacks)

1/3 c oat flour
1/3 c whole wheat pastry flour
1/4 c finely chopped walnuts or pecans
1/3 c dark brown sugar
1 T cinnamon
1/4 tsp sea salt
1/2 teaspoon baking powder
1 c finely chopped dates
2 egg whites beaten

Preheat oven 350 degrees. Lightly oil 8 "square pan. (I use spectrum organic no chemical) combine all ingredients except for the beaten egg whites. Add the whites into mix, stir just until blended, spoon batter into prepared pan. Bake 25 minutes, don't over bake. Cool before cutting into 24 little bite size squares.

Note: Seriously my clients loved this one! Each bite has 65 calories 1 g fat 2 g fiber 2 g protein 14 grams carbs (energy)

AMAZING TREAT OF A COOKIE

(not low fat)

2 C butter soft

1 c raw sugar

1.5 c brown sugar

2 eggs + 3 egg whites (or 4 large eggs)

2 tsp. Real vanilla

3 Cup king Arthur white whole wheat flour

3 cups old fashioned oats

2 tsp. baking powder

2 tsp. baking soda

1 T cinnamon

1 dark chocolate very good quality chocolate bar (Lindt is my favorite)

1 C dark chocolate chips

Preheat oven 350 degrees. Combine butter, sugars, eggs, vanilla, and shave the chocolate bar into this mixture once its mixed. In large food processor combine oats and flour, b. soda and Baking powder, cinnamon. Pulse to combine. (May need to do in 2 split processes) combine the dry into the wet and then add the chocolate chips. Stir and use a cookie scoop to assure cookies are uniform.

Note: This cookie has been a favorite during holidays, birthdays and a special treat at parties. For 20 years friends and family ask for them! I promised when I write a cookbook I would give the recipe out. They freeze really well and can be taken out 30 minute before serving.

HIGH FIBER BREAKFAST COOKIE

in large bowl combine
3/4 c brown sugar
1 stick soft butter
1/2 c unsweetened apple sauce
1/3 c raw cane sugar
1 whole organic egg + 2 egg whites
2 tsp vanilla

In another large bowl:
1 1/2 c whole wheat pastry flour
3/4 c unprocessed raw bran wheat
2 T cinnamon
1 tsp fresh ginger
1 tsp baking soda
A pinch sea salt
1/4 c 5 grain bobs red mill plus flax cereal
1/2 c dried bing cherries
1/2 c pumpkin seeds

Mix the dry into the wet and combine. Using a cookie scoop that will allow you to make 24 cookies, Bake at 375 degrees for approx 8-10 min. Don't overcook.

Health note; it's impossible to make a good tasting baked good eliminating all butter, however cutting back more than 1/2 of what your typical cookie recipe calls for saves you 800 calories per batch!

Each cookie: 70 calories, 2.5 g fiber   4 grams of fat but only 1 saturated

Note: to encourage your children to enjoy keeping their little intestinal system clean, add a little dark chocolate chips!

EASY SUMMER TIME SNACK

1/2 C fresh sweet Cantaloupe
2 T good quality Feta or Goat cheese
2 T finely chopped walnuts
1 T fresh chopped Basil

Place on a plate!

224 calories and 2 G fiber

MAIN DISHES

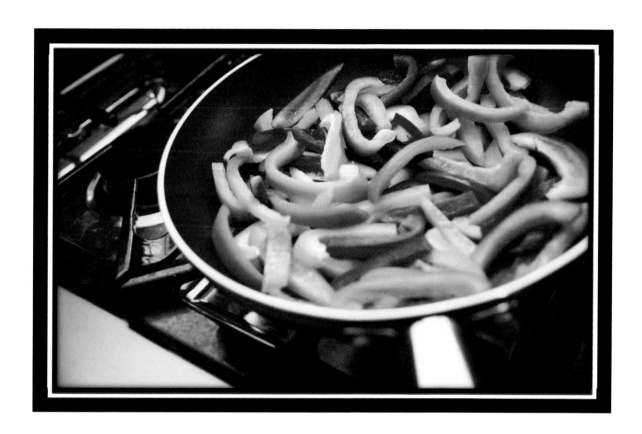

ROASTED RED PEPPER SAUCE

1 Jar of Roasted Red peppers drained
3 cloves garlic
2 sun dried tomatoes
3 Tablespoons extra virgin olive oil
1/3 c good quality Grated Parmesan cheese
1 Tablespoon balsamic vinegar

Place all ingredients in a food processor and pulse until smooth

Note: using roasted garlic gives it more flavor. Great on grilled chicken breast, burgers and even used on a loaf of toasted Italian bread.

GUILT FREE BAKED ROTINI PASTA

1 cup dry whole wheat Rotini or other pasta shape
1 cup whipped 1% fat cottage cheese
1 Tbsp. salt free seasoning
1 large zucchini washed and shredded
1 16 oz Roasted organic Tomatoes chopped (Mheir brand)
1/2 cup reduced Fat shredded Mozzarella cheese
1 handful of Fresh chopped Basil

Cook pasta as directed on Box. In the meantime in a nice serving/baking dish, combine the cottage cheese, seasoning, basil, roasted tomatoes, and fresh basil. Then add the zucchini, gently stir to combine and top with the Mozzarella cheese. Cover loosely with Foil and place in the oven on 350 for about 15 minutes. Remove foil and bake another 10 minutes to melt cheese until its bubbly.

Note: Makes 4 healthy portions (3 larger portions) Calories per serving of 4- 250 grams of protein 24 grams fiber 4 grams fat 2 grams carbohydrates. High fiber energy 30 grams.

TURKEY CUTLET WITH ZUCCHINI AND SWEET POTATO

(Easy as 1-2-3)

Two 4 oz slices turkey cutlets, pounded thin
A spritz of extra virgin olive oil or spectrum canola
Fresh lemon and zest
Two medium zucchini washed and shredded in food processor
1 large peeled sweet potato shredded the same way
1 Tablespoon spicy black bean spread (Trader Joes)
2 T no sugar added salsa hot or mild
2 T low sodium feta

Add turkey cutlets to a hot skillet that has been coated with oil, squeeze fresh lemon juice on them right away, they cook fast so flip after two minutes and squeeze lemon juice again on the cutlet, this time add 1 tbsp zest as well and cook for about 2 min. Remove from heat and place into serving dish. Sauté the shredded zucchini and sweet potato in the same pan with turkey cutlet juices for about 2 min. Add a dash of sea salt and pepper. Top the cutlet with the zucchini and sweet potato shreds. Place 1 tbsp. spicy black bean dip on top each cutlet and sprinkle with 1 T each Feta cheese. Serves 2 people. Calories 280 fiber 4 grams fat 8 grams

Note: If you use sweet potato, which I prefer, at the end of sautéing, add a dash of cinnamon or nutmeg and 1/4 tsp. honey before plating. If you use white potato the black pepper and feta are enough.

EXTRA LEAN ENCHILADA

Santa Fe whole grain high fiber wrap
1 lb extra lean ground turkey breast 1% fat
1/2 block Cabot 50% reduced fat sharp cheddar cheese
2 jars Enchilada sauce
1 small can green chilis
Chopped sweet red yellow peppers and onion about 1 c total

Spray large sauté pan with organic spectrum or 365 brand spray (no nitrates) cook meat first, adding onion and peppers to the mix about 1/2 way thru Cooking. Add the green chili's with juice and 1/2 cup shredded cheese to the mix, then add one jar Enchilada sauce to meat mixture. (Save the other jar for the topping as well as 1/2 c of the shredded cheese.) Lay out the tortillas and pour 1/4 c Enchilada sauce mixture first on the bottom of oblong dish to prevent sticking, than put 1/4 c mixture into the center of each tortilla, rolling into a tubular shape or you can cut the corners off and roll into a square. Once you've wrapped 5 you will drizzle the other jar of sauce on top. Sprinkle with remaining shredded cheese.

Bake 375 degree oven for about 10 minutes until cheese melts

Per Enchilada: calories 285 Fat: 5 g Carbs.: 16 grams of high fiber carbs Fiber 7 grams

Note: This dish can be made also with boiled chicken breast. Either way it's a healthy, filling, and quick meal for the family. You would simply add a dark green vegetable or salad to balance out your meal.

ONE GOOD CUP OF TURKEY CHILI

1 lb lean ground turkey breast

1 lb 7% fat turkey breast

1 c chopped sweet bell peppers red yellow and green

1/2 c chopped sweet Vidalia onion (use red if you can't find Vidalia)

2 cloves garlic chopped

1 small can green chili's

1 cup no sugar added salsa hot or medium heat

1 large can organic Roasted tomatoes chopped

2 T chili powder

1 T cumin

1 Can drained black beans

1 can drained kidney beans

1 Tbsp honey

2 Tbsp. Fresh lime juice

1 container of organic low sodium chicken broth

In a large pot add 1 tsp. olive oil to cook the garlic, onion, and peppers first. Then, add both packages of ground turkey and stir until done. Add tomatoes, salsa, broth, drained beans, and then all spices. Cover and cook on low to med. heat about 1 hour. Then add the honey and lime juice. Stir well and cook another 10 min. makes approx. 8-10 servings each serving is 250 calories * 2 grams fat * 28 grams protein

CHICKEN BREAST TOPPED WITH ROMA TOMATO

Organic chicken breast pounded thin (1 for each person)
1 T olive oil
1/3 c olive oil to marinade
Juice of 1 lime squeezed with the zest
1 T balsamic vinegar
1 Tablespoon honey
Handful fresh basil leaves
2 Roma tomatoes

Place pounded chicken breast in storage bag with 1/3 c olive oil, lime juice, zest and 1t balsamic vinegar. Leave in refrigerator for 1 hr (or up to 3 hrs.) Meanwhile have a stainless, oven proof skillet hot and add 1 T olive oil. Then add the chicken breast and sauté for about 5 min on one side. Flip and cook another 5 min. Have the oven on broil ready. Drizzle the honey over the chicken breast, sprinkle each chicken breast with 1 tsp. high quality parmesan cheese, slice the Roma tomatoes and layer on top of the chicken breast, sprinkle the fresh basil on top, place in oven in the middle rack for 2 min. to melt cheese. Let sit on stove to rest for 3-5 min.

Note: This dish is light, high in protein, low in fat, great tasting and goes well with a small portion of whole wheat pasta, roasted potatoes or mashed potatoes. Keeping the starch portion small and adding a great Dark Green vegetable will balance this meal out.

FAMOUS CHICKEN SALAD

(Secret ingredient!)

1 large package of lean chicken breast *about 6*
1/2 c canola Hellmann's light mayo
2 T good quality olive oil
1 large lemon squeezed over warm chicken and all of the zest
1 long stalk of celery cleaned and chopped small
1/4 C dried cranberries
1/4 c finely chopped Walnuts
1 Tbsp. black pepper
1 tsp sea salt
1 cup chopped sweet red grapes

The chicken needs to simmer for a very long time to tenderize it. Place in large pot with bay leaf, thyme, clove of garlic. Once it boils, turn it down, cover it lightly and let simmer about 2-3 hours. The chicken absorbs the flavor of the lemon and seasonings when it's still warm. Remove chicken from pot, and pull chicken breast apart with 2 forks so, it's more shredded rather than cut into pieces.

Mix mayo, olive oil, lemon juice, zest, black pepper and salt in large bowl. Pour over the top of the chicken. Mix the wet ingredients in well, and add a tad more light mayo if you feel it's necessary but, remember this is a healthier version of your typical chicken salad. Add the dried cranberries, celery, grapes & walnuts, a touch more pepper and stir well. Refrigerate.

Note: This is a family favorite we have a lot during summer outings. It's easy for entertaining as well. Its great on top of a green salad, or for making a sandwich (using "Arnold high fiber Flat bread" is a better choice for sandwiches) and it stays good for up to 4-5 days. My clients love this one!

LIGHT ON FAT HIGH IN PROTEIN TURKEY BURGER

1 lb extra lean ground turkey breast 1% fat

1/3 c greek 0% fat yogurt

1 thinly sliced stalk of celery

2 heaping Tablespoons Oat bran or oatmeal

2 egg whites

1 T black pepper

1 tsp sea salt

1 oz crumbled goat cheese or feta

1/4 c chopped fresh basil and parsley

2 T extra virgin olive oil

Mix all the ingredients together. Form little handful size patties to make burgers. You should get about 5-6. Place onto broil pan and in middle of the oven. They cook fast...after 5 minutes on one side flip and broil the other side for about 6-7 minutes. Calories per burger alone: 150 protein 16 grams carbs 1 gram fat 2 grams healthy fats

Note: I play with this all of the time adding slivered avocado on top, roasted pepper sauce you will find in the book under main meal because you can add it to anything, fresh sliced tomato, onion, etc. having a burger between a bun is heaven but often empty calories when speaking of bread. Try it on Arnold Flat rounds 100 calories per and up to 8 grams of additional fiber.

TURKEY BURGER THAT WONT LET YOU DOWN!

1 lb turkey breast ground
1/2 c. greek yogurt 0% fat
1 thinly sliced celery stalk
Dash of pepper and sea salt
1/3 C old fashioned oats
you can add hot sauce here, any spices you wish without sodium
Fresh rosemary chopped, oregano dash

Place approx 6 burgers on broiler pan.
Broil and watch closely On the middle rack 6 min. each side
*when you flip to 2nd side use 1/2 tsp. of a low sugar BB-Q sauce to top it and finish cooking.
Place 1/2 slice of fresh low fat cheese keep it light
Remove from hot pan to serving dish.

Have several topping choices available to your guest.
1-guacamole
2-tomato
3-lettuce
4-salsa
5- Mustard, low sugar ketchup

You can eat this on top of a large green salad. or use Arnold Flat rounds whole wheat 100 calories for your roll.

Enjoy!
6 smaller burgers with Guacamole and without round 130 calories
6 smaller burgers with Guacamole and with flat round 230 calories
(Or you can make 4 larger burgers for 180 calories without round)

CHICKEN BREAST MEATLOAF

Base:
One 6 oz can of no salt added tomato paste
1/4 c low sodium chicken stock
1 clove garlic chopped fine even better is roasted
1/4 c fresh chopped basil
1 T oregano
1/4 tsp sea salt
1 lb lean 1% fat ground chicken breast
1/2 c shredded zucchini
1/4 c liquid just whites all egg whites

Topping:
2 T ketchup
1/4 tsp dried mustard
1 T brown sugar
2 thin slices Best life approved Turkey bacon

Combine base ingredients; shape into a glass oblong pan or meatloaf pan. Have your turkey bacon already cooked and drying on paper towel. Combine the ketchup, dried mustard and brown sugar. Cover the top of meatloaf with this mix and lay the turkey bacon on top.
Bake 350 for approx. 35-45 minutes. Serves 8, each serving 200 calories
18 grams protein 7 grams fat 3 grams fiber

Note: my husband loves having this leftover on his sandwich for lunch the next day!

SIMPLE EASY WRAPS

"Smart & Delicious" brand low carb high fiber Tortillas (7 grams fiber) 13 oz
1 spray spectrum canola
1/2 c organic broccoli slaw
2.6 oz starkist light tuna or albacore
1 Tablespoon Guacamole
1 Tbsp. goat cheese or feta

Spray hot griddle with canola spectrum and place the wrap inside keeping heat medium to low. Quickly layer onto the tortilla, the tuna, broccoli slaw, guacamole, and cheese. Keep the cheese very light. Wrap each end over each other and flip it so the other side can get toasted.

Calories 205 Protein: 29 grams fiber:9 grams carbs: 10 grams

Note: The tortilla comes in 2 sizes. This recipe is using the smaller 36 calories - there is a larger one 100 calories and fiber is 12 grams. Keep it small, enjoy and know you will be eating again soon. You can make this in 5 minutes and get in a clean high fiber meal.

CHICKEN WRAP

(another easy simply done wrap)

3 oz left over boiled chicken breast shredded or grilled
Smart & delicious high fiber wrap
Broccoli slaw 1/2 c
Guacamole 1 T
1 triangle laughing cow light Swiss

In a hot griddle sprayed with spectrum canola oil, place wrap and quickly spread the soft laughing cow light cheese over bottom, layer the shredded or grilled chicken breast, broccoli slaw, and guacamole. Then wrap the ends over each other. Flip the wrap in pan to toast the other side.

Calories 195 Protein:19 grams Fat:2 grams Fiber:9 grams carbs (high fiber) 12 grams

WHOLE WHEAT PASTA WITH CHICKEN AND EXTRA TREAT

16 oz Barilla Plus whole wheat pasta
8- washed and center seeds cleaned out Roma Tomatoes
One 14.5 oz can Fire roasted crushed tomatoes Muir Glenn brand
1/2 C good quality Parmesan cheese
1 handful Fresh basil
1 T fresh oregano
1 whole chicken breast that has already been boiled and shredded w/ a fork
10 mini Aidells Chicken & apple Sausage (no msg no hormones)
2 cloves fresh garlic

Boil pasta as directed on box. Meanwhile in food processor add garlic, basil, oregano, and 2 T olive oil. chop and add the Roma and canned Fire roasted tomatoes. Place the chicken & apple sausage in the oven in 400 degrees for about 10 min. Turning 1/2 way. The chicken breast can be from a previous night of you making chicken salad, or other dish and keeping one out for this night making it quick. Place 1/2 c of the sauce on bottom of 8x11 dish, add pasta sprinkle with 1/2 cheese, add the meat, top with rest of sauce and cheese. Bake on 350 for 30 min.

Note: This recipes calories will vary depending on brand of pasta, and how much cheese you use but I assure you serving 6-7 people your intake will be about 350 calories. You should have a green salad to balance out your meal. I have added spinach to this pasta and it still is quite enjoyable.

LENTILS WITH GREENS

Tru Roots Organic sprouted green lentils (fresh market) entire package
2 large bunches of Rainbow or green Swiss chard
1 link chopped small chicken apple sausage *for vegetarian leave out*
1 Tbsp olive oil
1 clove garlic minced
1 Tbsp. good quality Parmesan cheese
Dash of Tabasco optional
3 cups low sodium chicken broth or Vegetable broth

Cook tru Roots sprouted lentils as on package 5 min. They still hold nutritional value and fiber! Meanwhile in large stock pot with 1 T olive oil, add chopped chicken apple sausage and garlic, sauté for 5 min. Add the broth and bring to a simmer. Meanwhile chop the chard into bite size pieces, wash well and add the chard to the pot. Cook for about 10 min.

Add a cup of greens to a plate and sprinkle with a little parmesan cheese. Place a 1/4- 1/2 cup cooked lentils on top and if you wish a dash of Tabasco.

Serves 4 -Calories per serving 400 which includes the chicken apple sausage 17 grams fiber, 30 grams protein

Note: For Vegetarians you can use soy based sausage or no meat at all however it does add flavor and protein.

POWER OF FITNESS QUICHE

1 whole slice Eziekel bread in food processor, pulse chop until tiny bits
1 pt organic egg whites
2 whole organic eggs
dash sea salt
dash pepper
dash cayenne pepper
1 whole sweet red pepper
2 small or 1 large zucchini
1/2 c finely shredded light Swiss or Guyere' cheese

In a deep dish rubber muffin cup tray, spray bottom quickly w/ spectrum canola spray, place 1 T. of the Eziekel crumbs on the bottom of each. In food processor combine egg whites, eggs, salt, pepper, cayenne. Once combined, pour all into a small bowl. Back in food processor shred the zucchini and sweet red pepper. (I have used jar Roasted peppers rinse too) pour that into the egg mix and also add the shredded cheese. Stir and scoop out 1/4-1/2 C of egg mixture into each muffin on top of the crumbs.

Bake 20 minutes 375. Don't over cook but all ovens vary so watch closely. Makes 5-6 Regular size Quiche- Calories 150 Protein 8 grams fiber 3 grams

Note: making little bite size is great too but, they tend to be more difficult to get out of pan without breaking. You can eat this with a salad or cup of soup for a meal or have at Breakfast. Make ahead and keep in the refrigerator for up to 3 days. Heat for 30 seconds to warm.

BRAISED GREENS AND SWEET POTATOES

2 med. small sweet onion
2 cloves garlic minced
3 medium sweet potatoes peeled and cut into 16 equal pieces
3 c. vegetable stock
4 cups turnips, kale, or other dark leafy Greens washed stems discarded
1/4 tsp cayenne pepper
1 1/2 T cider vinegar
1 T Fresh thyme
sea salt and ground black pepper
2 T EVOO (extra virgin olive oil)

In med size pot over med heat, add olive oil and onions and cook 3 min. next add cayenne pepper and garlic and cook 1 minute. Season lightly and stir to combine. Add stock, vinegar and thyme. Bring to a simmer and add chopped greens and sweet potatoes. Cook until greens and potatoes are tender. The Potato will thicken the stock and make it slightly sweet.

my clients loved this dish and make it all of the time

WHAT TO DO WITH A WHOLE CHICKEN

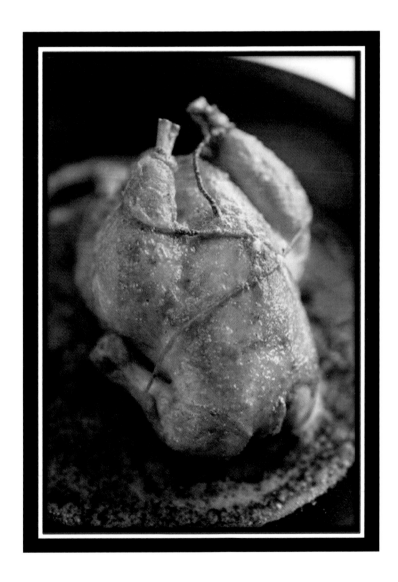

What to do with a whole chicken?
Other than roasting of course......Make 3 meals out of one whole chicken!
Start with a very large soup pot. Wash chicken and take the bag of chicken liver out.

CHICKEN SOUP

Place Chicken in a large pot to make a soup broth.
Add 2 whole carrots 2 stalks celery, 3 cloves garlic, 1 small sweet onion
Add a touch of sea salt and pepper.

Simmer for about 1.5-2 hours. You want the chicken to be falling off when you touch it.

Remove chicken from the stock and place in a large bowl to cool slightly so you can begin to remove meat. Drain your stock. (Divide into two portions so you can use for another recipe)

Keeping the pot hot add 1 tsp. olive oil fresh garlic clove chopped, 2 stalks fresh celery chopped 2 whole carrots chopped and add 1 can organic Cannellini beans, sauté for about 3 min.

Begin to pick off some of your chicken and add to the pot which is now turned down to low. Add a large bunch of cleaned and chopped kale. sauté for a minute and then add your stock back into the pot. (if you need more stock to make larger pot of soup use a low sodium chicken stock to add in)

I prefer to keep this low carb with only veggies and chicken however you can always add 1/2 c cooked orzo or brown rice to this soup.

*another good option is to avoid pasta, and add cut up sweet potato or butternut squash instead. You would add this to the soup when you add the kale and it will be your starch. Any starch that isn't man touched is best for your body.

Throw in a handful of fresh parsley at end if you have it on hand and sprinkle with 1/2 tsp. parmesan cheese right at serving

Enjoy.

MEXICAN DISH

(meal #2 more chicken left?)

Place the white meat part of chicken in an oblong dish (this can be done the next day after its been Refrigerated)

Pour a 1/2 can of washed black beans over chicken add 1 small can roasted chopped tomatoes

Add 3 T fresh or no sugar added salsa on top

You can add olives here as well

Place foil over it and bake for about 15 min. on 375

Sprinkle low fat cheddar cheese on top about 1/2 c total and bake for another 5-8 min. uncovered.

This goes great with a green salad.

This meal feeding 4 people will give you approx 330 cal. and 8 grams fiber per serving and only 3 grams fat. When using lean meats and no sugar added as well as low fat cheese you are saving yourself about 15 g fat.

CHICKEN POT PIE

(meal #3 one of my family favorites winter dish)

*truth be told its impossible to make a chicken pot pie that taste good without adding a little touch of fat but we've leaned this one out for you.

In a large pot sauté a clove of garlic in 1 T olive oil and 1 T unsalted butter 2 stalks of chopped carrot and celery sauté for about 5 min. on med. heat

Add to this pot your other 1/2 of chicken stock (again adding low sodium stock from carton if needed but you should only have about 2 cups total)

cube 1 large peeled sweet potato
cube 2 small to medium size Yukon gold potatoes
Then add the potatoes to the pot with the rest of your cut up chicken from the original recipe *about 2 cups meat
Add 1/2 bag organic corn, edamame, green bean mixture (trader joes)

Simmer for about 20 in. on low

In a small skillet add 1/2 tsp. unsalted butter melt and add 2 T either whole wheat pastry flour or oat flour. Use a whisk and whisk fast to smooth it out. Immediately pour 1/2 c nonfat condensed milk into it and continue to stir to a thick smooth consistency. Next ladle in 1/4 c broth and whisk again pouring it all into your larger pot.

Simmer another 10 min.

Using a large ladle or spoon that has holes in it, scoop the vegetable portion into 4-5 serving bowls. I like to make 5 to keep portion smaller. Make sure you use an oven proof bowl that hold about 1/2 -2 c. without overflowing.

Once you've portioned out the mixture than you ladle the broth into each bowl. lastly using a Pillsbury pie crust roll it out super thin! The thin means less calories but still having a nice texture and crunch to your crust.

Using one of the rolls of crust cut into 2" strips lying across each bowl and then across the opposite directions.

You can just cover the bowl completely and pinch sides, however make sure you really use thin crust as you will be adding calories to your end result.

Bake about 10 min. on 375. Be very careful when removing from oven and let sit for about 5-10 min. as it will be piping a hot!

By following this recipe you save yourself about 400 calories and 30 grams of fat based on a typical pot pie. This pot pie feeding 5 has approx. 300 calories and 7 g fat.

PUMP UP WITH BEVERLY

"You've Got the Power, Use It!"

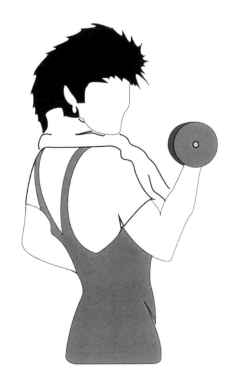

POWER PROTEIN PANCAKE

3/4 c old fashions oats
2 egg whites + 1 whole organic egg
1 T cinnamon
1/2 c 1% fat whipped cottage cheese
1/2 scoop high quality vanilla protein powder (ump)

Heat griddle to med. spray organic spectrum non chemical canola on pan to prevent sticking. Puree all ingredients in blender and pour 1/4 cup into griddle (non stick is important) flip after 1 minute and cook for another 30 seconds.

Serving size 2 pancakes calories: 300 protein: 26 grams Fat. 1 gram carbohydrates: (energy) 10 grams

Note: Beverly ultimate muscle protein is my favorite www.bodybuildingworld.com topping this pancake with 1 Tablespoon natural nut butter will balance the breakfast with a healthy fat adding 90 calories and 7 grams protein

POWER ENERGY BALLS

(Quick healthy grab and go snacks)

15 pitted dates
2 T natural nut butter
1 scoop Beverly UMP vanilla (www.bodybuildingworld.com)

Simply chop dates first in food processor, add nut butter of your choice and Beverly protein powder. Puree until you get a thick smooth paste. *you will have a few date chunks and that is ok* Take about 1/2 tsp. out at a time with clean dry hands make tiny ball and place on wax paper to set. Make about 15-20 ball depending on your size. I like to keep them small.

Each little bite size Power energy ball has calories:30 protein: 2.5 grams fiber 1 gram fat 1/2 gram healthy fat

Note: another favorite of clients! Using as a quick jolt when on a long run or workout. They freeze well so, you can double up on recipe. Keep in the refrigerator up to a week (if they last that long!)

BANANA COCONUT MINI CHOCOLATE CHIP CUPCAKE

(Beverly pumped protein)

1 c oat flour
1/2 teaspoon baking soda
1/2 teaspoon baking powder
1 small ripe banana
1/3 c organic brown sugar
2 egg whites
1/3 c greek 0% fat plain yogurt
1/3 c flaked coconut
1/3 c sunspire organic 65% dark chocolate chips (mini if you can find them
1 scoop chocolate Beverly muscle provider (www.bodybuildingworld.com)

Spray a mini muffin pan or use the rubber non stick ones. Combine in the food processor the banana, yogurt, brown sugar, egg whites, coconut and puree. In a large bowl combine the flour, baking soda, baking powder, chocolate chips and Beverly chocolate muscle provider. Combine the wet ingredients into the dry and stir well. Use a small cookie scoop to make it easier to get into the mini muffin cups.

Bake at 350 8-10 min. watch closely so they don't dry out. Makes 20 mini muffins *each mini muffins: calories: 56 fiber: 2 grams Protein: 2.6 carbs: 6 grams

Note: I prefer not to use paper muffin fillers. Also, the muffins can be drizzled with a thin glaze of organic melted dark chocolate for a real treat.

CHOCOLATE POWER OF FITNESS PROTEIN BARS

1 scoop Beverly chocolate muscle provider (www.bodybuildingworld.com)
1/2 c cashew nut butter organic *you can use any natural nut butter*
30 pitted dates
5 Prunes
1/2 c organic Agave *use honey if you don't have agave*
1/4 c raw oatbran
1 T chai seeds
1/2 c raw unsalted pumpkin seeds
1/2 c organic 65% sunspire chocolate chips
1 egg white (just whites)

In food processor add all of the ingredients except pumpkin seeds and chocolate chips. Pulse/chop and continue until it begins to look wet and combines. Add the pumpkin seeds and chips and quickly pulse to blend. Use wax paper and dump the mixture into a 8x8 square pan. Press it all down to form a solid square. Place in the refrigerator for an hour or more. Then cut into 20 bars.

Each bar: Calories: 80 Protein: 2.5 grams fiber: 1.5 grams carbs: 4 grams

Note: stays fresh in refrigerator for up to a week. You can individually wrap them and freeze or just have them to grab as a quick treat.

PUMP UP THE MUSCLE WITH BEVERLY

(Quick fix tried and true)

1/2 c Friendship all natural 1% fat Whipped Cottage cheese
1 T natural nut butter *your choice cashew, almond or peanut*
1/2 scoop Beverly ultimate muscle protein chocolate or Vanilla

Mix together the cottage cheese, nut butter and Beverly UMP powder. Stir well and enjoy.

240 calories 30 grams high protein! carbs: 5 grams

Note: This may seem like a crazy combo but, I promise it is worth trying. Several years ago while on vacation I just came back from a workout, usually eating eggs but it was hot and my creativity put these 3 ingredients in a bowl and yummy!! It's a quick fix full of calcium protein and healthy fat.

HIGH FIBER BANANA BRAN COOKIE

(pump up with Beverly)

1/4 c raw sugar
1 stick soft butter
1 large organic egg
1 T cinnamon
2 small ripe bananas
1/2 c unsweetened organic applesauce
1/4 c raw oat bran
1 C finely chopped Kellogg's complete bran cereal flakes
1 scoop chia seeds (antioxidant rich and omega 3)
1/2 scoop Beverly UMP powder (optional for more protein to your cookie)
1/4 c raw unsalted pumpkin seeds
1/4 c sweet golden raisins
1 c whole wheat pastry flour

Combine in Food processor sugar, butter, egg, cinnamon, banana, and applesauce. In a large bowl combine oat bran, cereal flakes that have already been finely chopped, whole wheat flour, chia seeds, and Beverly protein powder (if using). Stir by hand the wet ingredients into the dry. Use a small cookie scoop and bake at 350 for 8-10 minutes on middle rack. Do not over bake. These cookies are best eaten the day of baking.

Makes 30 cookies. calories per cookie 48 protein with UMP 2.8 grams Fiber: 2 grams

Note: my background allows me to graze throughout the day, and this is a treat with a cup of Tea mid am. or afternoon. To encourage your children to get the fiber in add chocolate chips to this mix and your little ones will have no problem!

QUICK FIXINS

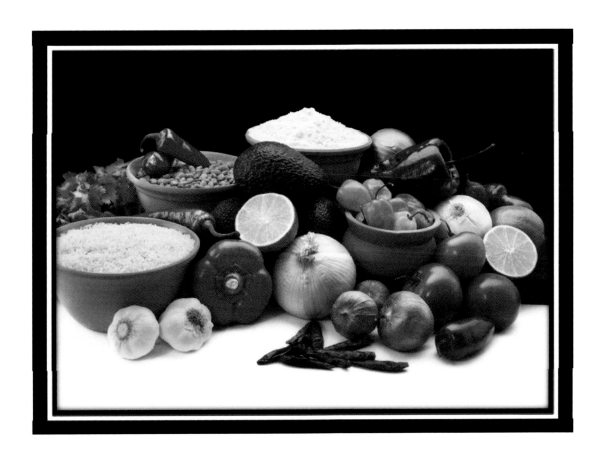

A FEW OF MY FAVORITES,

ALTHOUGH SOME MAY SEEM ODD,

I SUGGEST TRYING.

CRUNCH AND SATISFACTION PLEASE!

Kamut Puffed Agave sweetened rice cake (whole foods)
*only 30 calories for each

Top with 1 T natural nut butter (make sure it's all natural no added oils) and sprinkle with 1/2 scoop Chia seed *high in omega 3 and antioxidants

You'd be surprised at how satisfying this little treat is!

Calories; total 160
Fat: 4 - heart healthy fats
Fiber: 4 grams
protein: 5 grams

PROTEIN AND VEGGIES PLEASE!

Chicken and apple organic Wilshire Farm sausage (whole foods)
Fresh organic Baby spinach leaves
Pinch of either low sodium feta or goat cheese.

Spray the pan with one spritz or use only 1/4 tbsp. of olive oil
Remember these calories add up so best to use spay

Brown 1 link only of Wilshire farm chicken sausage for about 5 min.
Take it out and chop up into bite size

Spray pan one more time if needed only

Toss 2 large handfuls of baby spinach into hot pan and add the sausage back into pan. Remove from heat and top with 2 Tablespoons only of Feta or goat cheese.

Calories: 95 calories
Fat: 4.5 grams NO transfat
Protein: 7.5 grams

POTASSIUM TO PLEASE THE CRAMPS!

1 banana
Peel and top with 1 T nut butter
Sprinkle 1/2 scoop chia seed on top
Drizzle w/ 1/4 tbsp. honey

150 calories
Fat heart healthy 2.5 grams
Protein 2 grams
Fiber 4.5 grams
Again omega 3 antioxidants and potassium! can't beat it!

LUNCH ON THE RUN, OR AN EASY DINNER

I would never completely give up on fixes that help you make a healthy meal with a little help! The best advice is to boil organic chicken breast on your day off.

Simmer for at least 3 hrs. on low to allow tenderness. Keep it covered in the refrigerator for up to 4 days ready to toss into another dish!

Take Green Giant Immunity Blend frozen boxed Vegetables and microwave about 5 min.

While that is going, take 4 oz of your boiled chicken breast out and toss into a skillet just to get it warm. Drizzle with 1/4 tsp olive oil or better yet spray. Begin to chop some of the chicken with a spoon and add your immunity blend on top with all juices.

Simmer for about 3 min. and you've got a meal.

Calories: 190 (yes i want you to eat the entire box of vegetables)
Fat: 2.5 NO transfat
Carbs: 11 grams
Fiber 2 grams
Protein 21 grams.

HEAT AND EAT WRAP

This is one of my favorite quick lunches!!

Heat a skillet on medium heat. Spray with spectrum canola spray just once.

Lay flat in the pan:
1 light original wrap
Empty a chunk light tuna pouch in water down the center of wrap
Top with 1//3 of a fresh avocado sliced (portion control on this!)
Top with 1 c broccoli slaw (trader joes) right out of the bag no added mayo
Wrap the side over and flip so other side will get warm
Slice in 1/2 and enjoy!

Calories: 260
Protein: 29 grams
Fiber: 12 grams
Fat is healthy fat from avocado 3 grams

QUICK TUNA AVOCADO

(one of my favorites and works on a gluten free plan)

1 pouch light tuna (in water)
1 cup broccoli slaw
1/2 fresh cut avocado
1 Tbsp. pumpkin seeds
1 T extra virgin olive oil

On a plate simply layer all ingredients allowing the avocado, tuna and olive oil to moisten the broccoli slaw.
Enjoy either alone or with a few rice crackers.

Calories: 410 (keep in mind these calories are from your healthy fats)
Fiber: 6 grams
Protein: 23 grams
Fat:5 grams of monounsaturated .

Phytonutrients are believed to prevent many chronic diseases; therefore in this meal you should not be so concerned about the calories as they are good quality.

Note: during a detox when wheat, dairy, soy, gluten, are avoided this was very helpful and if you are really hungry you can add 1/4 c cooked brown rice to the dish.

TIPS FROM THE AUTHOR

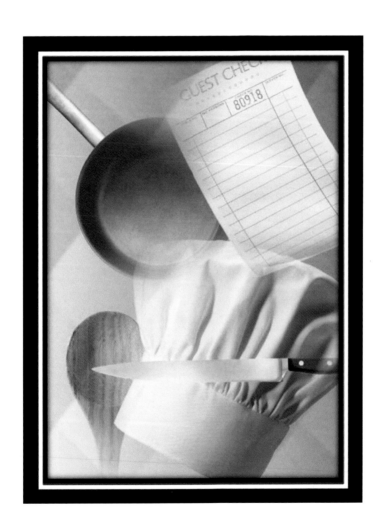

DID YOU KNOW TIDBITS:

I have found over the years that learning a bit of info about the foods you eat actually encourage you to either eat more of a good food or eat less of a bad one. For example, did you know:

<u>1 stick of butter alone has 800 calories!</u> (Most baking recipes call for 2 or more sticks; this is where you would substitute Greek yogurt or applesauce to replace some of that bad fat.

<u>Marinating Beef</u> in red wine before grilling significantly reduces Carcinogens.

<u>Dark chocolate</u> (70% cocoa or higher) is rich in Antioxidants and actually good for you in moderation. Flavonoids which help the lining of the Vessels expand and contract to improve blood flow.

<u>Blueberries & mint</u> make a great compliment for each other and blueberries alone have one of the highest purest antioxidants that fight age and disease.

<u>Papaya</u> is great for your skin, helps with sinus congestion and relieves bloating. One cup has only 55 calories. Its great with Greek yogurt or on salads.

<u>Frozen vegetables</u> can be just as nutritional as fresh when you can't purchase in season produce. They are flash frozen as soon as they are picked, which means they retain their value.

<u>Olive oil</u> is packed with monounsaturated fat and is great for your heart, However it packs 120 calories per Tablespoon, therefore "portion control" is important.

<u>Apples</u>: great snack, high in fiber, about 3 grams and only 70 calories

<u>Banana</u>: great in smoothies offering 3 g fiber and 100 calories. Helps eliminate cramps, full of potassium.

<u>Cherries</u>: Fresh about 27 give you 116 calories and 4 g fiber

<u>Grapes:</u> 1 cup 62 calories 1 g fiber
*keep in mind both of these have a natural sweetness when in season allowing you to satisfy your craving without added processing or additives.

<u>All Bran Buds and Fiber one Cereal</u> both pack a great punch when it comes to fiber. By simply adding 1/4 cup to your yogurt parfait or any baked item you have, even on top of salads for a great crunch, you get 13 grams of fiber which is 51% of your daily recommended fiber intake.

TRICKS TO ADD FLAVOR AND LOWER FAT:

Often times just making little changes in your recipe can save thousands of calories and fat which can lead to a significant weight loss in a year. Give some of these a try, Even with some of the recipes I have offered to you in this book.

Instead of using heavy cream or butter try cooking and then pureeing vegetables such as, cauliflower, carrots, sweet potato or butternut squash. Add to soups, pasta sauces that call for cream, and I have even done this for my chicken pot pie.

Instead of pouring oil (even though its healthy fat it's still fat) onto your vegetables when roasting, try using a purchased spray bottle and pouring olive oil into it for less oil in cooking. You can also steam your veggies first than place them on a grill after steaming with Ms. Dash or another no sodium seasoning for Great flavor!

Bake your fish instead of frying.

Bake your turkey meatballs first and then place them into pot of sauce to finish cooking.

When a recipe calls for heavy cream, try mixing plain fat free yogurt with low fat ricotta.

Another great idea is to puree fresh fruit adding only 1/2 tsp. organic biodynamic native sweetener (12 calories) whole foods- to 1 cup fruit then pour this mixture over top of angel food cake (low fat and does have sugar) or NO sugar added low fat vanilla ice cream. Now this is a treat!

EATING OUT SHOULD NOT BE OUT OF THE QUESTION:

Eating out can cause major havoc in the weight loss plan because our restaurants tend to add way too much salt to our meals and the portions are out of control! But you know that already so, here are a few places that I encourage my clients to try because I know they are aware of health concerns and cautious about the added fats, chemicals and sodium.

You can ask for your meals to be altered in any way to better fit your needs and you will never have a problem with your meal.

PUNKS BACKYARD GRILL

House salad with choice of 2 skewers. Ask for the dressing on the side. (I never use dressing but you can use 1/2 of the little cup)
1 steak skewer 157 calories 9 grams fat 18 grams protein 55 grams sodium
1 shrimp skewer 90 calories 1.5 g fat 17 grams protein 126 grams sodium

by adding the house salad with very little dressing you can make a satisfying meal high in protein, lower sodium than the average eating out meal and lower you can control your meal intake.

Another option at Punks but must order carefully asking for NO BBQ sauce and NO bread due to the roll being white and BBQ sauce having too much sugar.

Homemade Veggie burger NO bread, on top of grilled Asparagus salad NO flat bread either it has oil before grilling. Dressing on side. This veggie burger is by far the best I have ever had knowing Punks makes theirs from scratch from locally grown farms ingredients makes it worth trying.

RUBY TUESDAY

Tilapia meal easy on seasoning due to sodium, NO sauce, brown rice pilaf and broccoli steamed no oil.

This meal is very satisfying. Asking for it prepared healthier is easy to do, and it will save you many calories and loads of sodium taken off of your meal.

Eating out makes it difficult to lose weight if you choose to do so more than once per week. Give some of these easy recipes in my book a try, and you will see that time in the kitchen can be enjoyable, slowing down to enjoy your family knowing you are not only feeding yourself better but your family too.